BOOK TITLE

Pregnancy and Postpartum Fitness

SUBTITLE: Focusing on safe and effective exercises and nutrition during pregnancy and the postpartum period.

AUTHOR'S NAME

ERIC UROH

Dedication

3

To all the mothers embarking on the beautiful journey of pregnancy and postpartum, this eBook is dedicated to you. May it serve as a guiding light, offering support, encouragement, and inspiration as you prioritize your health and fitness during this transformative time. Your strength, resilience, and dedication to your well-being are truly admirable, and I hope this resource empowers you to thrive physically, mentally, and emotionally on your path to motherhood.

Pregnancy and Postpartum Fitness

Table Of Contents

5

Introduction:

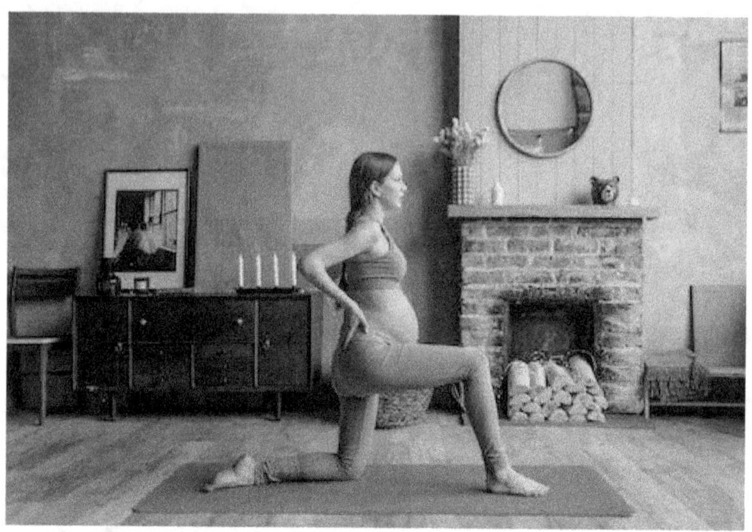

In the transformative journey of pregnancy and the postpartum period, prioritizing fitness is not just about staying active it's about nurturing your body and mind through this profound experience. Welcome to "Pregnancy and Postpartum Fitness," a comprehensive guide designed to support you in embracing the power of movement before, during, and after childbirth.

A. **Importance of Fitness During Pregnancy and Postpartum**:

Throughout the stages of pregnancy and into the postpartum period, maintaining a focus on fitness is crucial. Exercise not only helps to prepare the body for the physical demands of childbirth but also plays a significant role in promoting overall well-being. By incorporating safe and appropriate exercises, you can enhance your strength, endurance, and flexibility, laying the foundation for a smoother pregnancy, delivery, and recovery.

B. **The Physical and Emotional Benefits**:

The benefits of prenatal and postpartum fitness extend far beyond physical health. Engaging in regular exercise can boost mood, alleviate stress, and enhance sleep quality vital aspects of emotional well-being during this transformative time. By nurturing your body through movement, you cultivate a deeper connection with yourself and your growing baby, fostering a sense of empowerment and confidence as you navigate the journey of motherhood.

C. **Purpose and Scope of the Guide**:

This guide is a comprehensive resource crafted to provide you with the knowledge, tools, and support necessary to embark on a safe and effective fitness journey during pregnancy and beyond. From understanding the physiological changes your body undergoes to creating personalized exercise plans tailored to your needs, each chapter is designed to equip you with practical strategies and insights. Whether you're a first-time mother or welcoming a new addition to your family, this guide is here to empower you to prioritize your health and well-being throughout the miraculous journey of pregnancy and postpartum recovery.

As we delve into the chapters ahead, we'll explore topics ranging from understanding the intricacies of pregnancy-related changes to crafting effective exercise routines and nurturing your body through proper nutrition and self-care practices. Additionally, we'll discuss the importance of seeking professional support and sharing inspiring real-life stories from individuals who have embarked on their own pregnancy and postpartum fitness journeys.

Get ready to embark on a transformative adventure one that celebrates the strength, resilience, and beauty of the human body. Together, let's embrace the power of fitness to support you through every step of your pregnancy and postpartum experience.

9

Chapter 1: Understanding Pregnancy and Postpartum Fitness

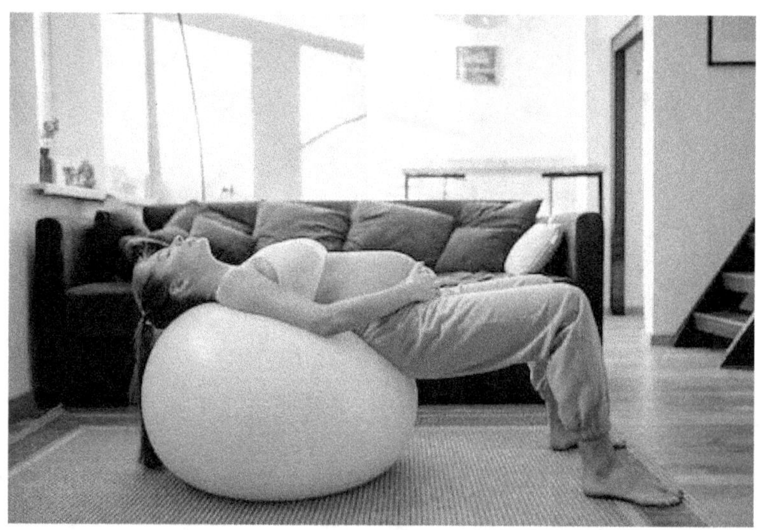

A. The Changes Your Body Goes Through:

1. Hormonal Shifts:

During pregnancy, your body undergoes significant hormonal changes to support the growth and development of your baby. Hormones such as estrogen and progesterone increase dramatically, influencing various physiological processes. These hormonal shifts can affect your mood, energy levels, and metabolism. Additionally, hormones like relaxing contribute to the relaxation of ligaments and joints, preparing your body for childbirth but also increasing the risk of injury during exercise.

2. **Musculoskeletal Changes**:

As your pregnancy progresses, your body experiences musculoskeletal changes to accommodate the growing fetus and prepare for childbirth. Your center of gravity shifts forward, leading to alterations in posture and balance. The increased weight of the uterus can strain the back and pelvis, leading to discomfort and potential musculoskeletal issues. Additionally, the abdominal muscles may separate (diastasis recti) to make room for the expanding uterus, impacting core strength and stability.

3. **Cardiovascular Adaptations**:

Pregnancy places significant demands on the cardiovascular system to support both the mother and the developing fetus. Blood volume increases, and the heart rate rises to meet the body's increased oxygen and nutrient needs. Hormonal changes also affect blood vessel function, leading to changes in blood pressure. These cardiovascular adaptations help ensure adequate oxygen and nutrients reach the placenta and support fetal growth and development.

B. **Safety Considerations**:

1. **Medical Clearance**:

Before starting any exercise program during pregnancy or postpartum, it's essential to obtain medical clearance from your healthcare provider. Your doctor or midwife can assess your health status, any pre-existing medical conditions, and potential pregnancy-related complications to determine the safety of exercise. Medical clearance ensures that you can engage in physical activity safely and effectively, minimizing the risk of adverse outcomes for you and your baby.

2. **Prenatal and Postpartum Exercise Guidelines**:

Understanding and adhering to prenatal and postpartum exercise guidelines is crucial for promoting maternal and fetal health. Prenatal exercise guidelines typically recommend moderate-intensity aerobic activity and strength training exercises that focus on maintaining muscle tone and pelvic floor strength. Postpartum exercise guidelines emphasize gradual progression and the importance of pelvic floor rehabilitation to support recovery and prevent injury. It's essential to follow these guidelines carefully and modify exercises as needed to accommodate the changing needs of your body throughout pregnancy and postpartum.

3. **Common Pregnancy-related Conditions**:

Pregnancy can bring about various physiological changes and potential complications that may impact your ability to exercise safely. Common pregnancy-related conditions such as gestational diabetes, preeclampsia, and pelvic girdle pain (PGP) can affect your mobility and exercise tolerance. It's essential to be aware of these conditions and work closely with your healthcare provider to manage them effectively while staying active. Additionally, understanding warning signs and symptoms that may indicate the need to modify or discontinue exercise is crucial for ensuring the safety of both you and your baby.

By gaining a deeper understanding of the changes your body undergoes during pregnancy and postpartum, as well as prioritizing safety considerations, you can embark on a fitness journey that supports your health and well-being throughout this transformative experience.

Chapter 2: Prenatal Exercise

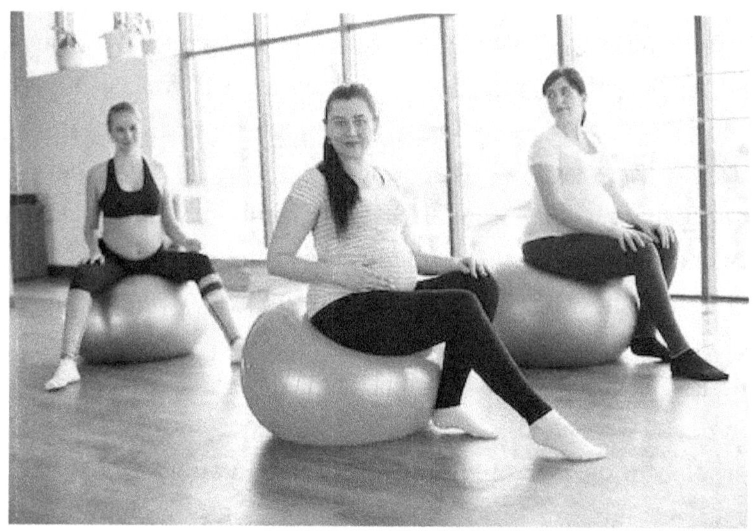

Pregnancy is a unique journey that presents both opportunities and challenges and incorporating regular exercise into your prenatal routine can have numerous benefits for both you and your baby. In this chapter, we'll explore the benefits of prenatal exercise, different types of exercises suitable for pregnancy, how to create a personalized prenatal exercise plan, essential nutrition, and hydration tips, and address common concerns and myths surrounding exercise during pregnancy.

A. **Benefits of Exercise During Pregnancy**:

Regular exercise during pregnancy offers a myriad of benefits for both the expectant mother and her developing baby:

- Improved cardiovascular health: Aerobic exercise helps maintain cardiovascular fitness, promoting efficient blood circulation and oxygen delivery to both the mother and fetus.

- Enhanced mood and mental well-being: Exercise releases endorphins, which can alleviate stress, reduce anxiety, and enhance mood during pregnancy.

- Better sleep quality: Engaging in physical activity can help alleviate pregnancy-related discomfort and improve sleep quality.

- Reduced risk of gestational diabetes and preeclampsia: Exercise has been shown to reduce the risk of developing gestational diabetes and preeclampsia, two common pregnancy-related complications.

- Enhanced muscular strength and endurance: Strength training exercises help maintain muscle tone, improve posture, and prepare the body for the physical demands of childbirth.

- Preparation for labor and delivery: Certain exercises, such as prenatal yoga and pelvic floor exercises, can help strengthen the muscles used during labor and promote optimal fetal positioning.

B. **Types of Prenatal Exercise**:

1. **Aerobic Exercise**:

Aerobic exercises such as walking, swimming, and cycling are excellent choices for prenatal fitness as they are low-impact and help improve cardiovascular health without placing excessive stress on the joints.

2. **Strength Training**:

Strength training exercises using body weight, resistance bands, or light weights can help maintain muscle tone and strength during pregnancy. Focus on compound exercises that target multiple muscle groups, such as squats, lunges, and modified push-ups.

3. **Yoga and Pilates**:

Prenatal yoga and Pilates focus on gentle stretching, strengthening, and relaxation techniques that can help alleviate pregnancy-related discomfort, improve flexibility, and promote mental well-being.

4. **Low-Impact vs. High-Impact Exercises**:

Low-impact exercises, such as walking and swimming, are generally safe and comfortable for most pregnant women, especially those with joint pain or pelvic floor issues. High-impact exercises, such as running or jumping, may be suitable for some women earlier in pregnancy but may need to be modified or avoided as pregnancy progresses.

C. **Creating a Prenatal Exercise Plan**:

1. **Setting Goals**:

Establish clear and realistic fitness goals based on your individual needs, preferences, and fitness level. Consider factors such as your current health status, stage of pregnancy, and any pregnancy-related complications.

2. **Finding Suitable Classes or Trainers**:

Look for prenatal exercise classes or certified fitness trainers with experience and expertise in working with pregnant women. Choose activities that are safe, enjoyable, and appropriate for your fitness level and stage of pregnancy.

3. **Safe Exercise Techniques**:

Practice proper form and technique during exercises to minimize the risk of injury. Avoid activities that involve lying flat on your back or require rapid changes in direction, and listen to your body's cues to avoid overexertion.

D. **Nutrition and Hydration Tips**:

Maintaining a balanced diet and staying hydrated are essential components of a healthy prenatal exercise routine. Aim to consume nutrient-dense foods that provide essential vitamins, minerals, and macronutrients to support both you and your baby's health. Drink plenty of water before, during, and after exercise to prevent dehydration and ensure optimal hydration levels.

E. **Addressing Common Concerns and Myths**:

Dispelling common concerns and myths surrounding exercise during pregnancy is essential for promoting a safe and healthy prenatal fitness routine. Address misconceptions such as the fear of harming the baby, the belief that exercise should be avoided altogether, and the misconception that pregnancy is a time to "eat for two." Educate yourself about the benefits of exercise during pregnancy and consult with your healthcare provider to address any specific concerns or questions you may have.

By incorporating safe and appropriate exercises into your prenatal routine, you can optimize your physical and mental well-being throughout pregnancy, prepare your body for childbirth, and lay the foundation for a smooth postpartum recovery. Remember to listen to your body, prioritize safety, and enjoy the many benefits that prenatal exercise has to offer.

Chapter 3: Postpartum Fitness

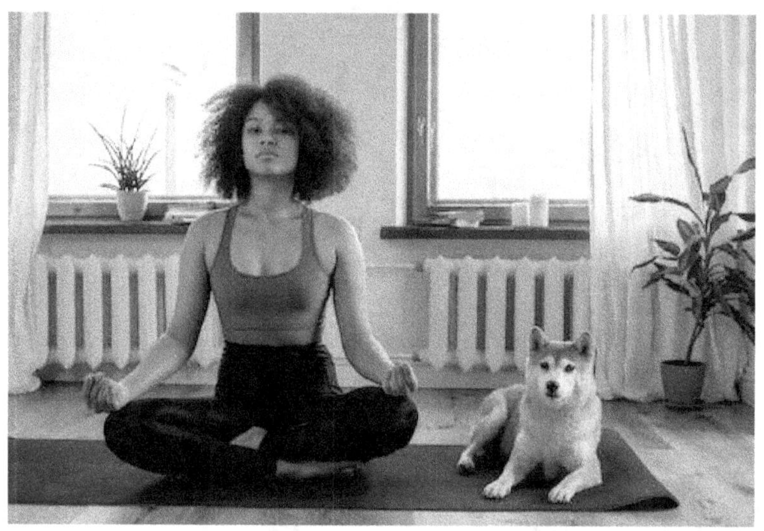

As you transition into the postpartum period, focusing on your physical and emotional well-being becomes paramount. This chapter delves into what to expect during the postpartum period, the importance of core and pelvic floor health, guidelines for safely returning to exercise, and strategies for embracing postpartum changes and prioritizing self-care.

A. **The Postpartum Period: What to Expect:**

1. **Physical Recovery**:

The postpartum period encompasses the weeks and months following childbirth, during which your body undergoes significant changes as it recovers from pregnancy and delivery. Physical recovery varies for each woman but may include healing from childbirth-related injuries, such as tears or episiotomies, and returning to pre-pregnancy levels of strength and mobility.

2. **Emotional Well-being**:

Alongside physical recovery, the postpartum period brings a range of emotions, from joy and fulfillment to anxiety and exhaustion. It's common to experience mood swings, postpartum blues, or even postpartum depression. Prioritizing emotional well-being and seeking support from loved ones and healthcare providers are crucial during this transitional period.

B. **The Importance of Core and Pelvic Floor Health**:

1. **Diastasis Recti**:

Diastasis recti is a common condition characterized by the separation of the abdominal muscles along the midline of the abdomen. This separation can lead to core weakness, lower back pain, and poor posture. Engaging in specific exercises to strengthen the deep core muscles and gradually closing the gap can aid in recovery.

2. **Pelvic Floor Dysfunction**:

Pregnancy and childbirth can weaken the pelvic floor muscles, leading to issues such as urinary incontinence, pelvic organ prolapse, and sexual dysfunction. Pelvic floor exercises, also known as Kegels, can help strengthen these muscles and alleviate symptoms of pelvic floor dysfunction.

C. **Gradual Return to Exercise**:

1. **Postpartum Exercise Guidelines**:

Gradually reintroducing exercise after childbirth is essential to allow your body time to heal and regain strength. Begin with gentle activities such as walking, pelvic floor exercises, and gentle stretching, gradually progressing to more strenuous exercises as your body allows. Listen to your body's cues and avoid pushing yourself too hard too soon.

2. **Post-Cesarean Section Considerations**:

If you've had a cesarean section, your recovery may take longer, and you may need to modify your exercise routine accordingly. Avoid high-impact activities and exercises that place excessive strain on the abdominal muscles until your incision has fully healed. Consult with your healthcare provider for personalized guidance on post-Cesarean exercise.

D. **Body Image and Self-Care**:

1. **Embracing Postpartum Changes**:

Pregnancy and childbirth bring about significant changes to your body, and it's essential to embrace and celebrate these changes as a testament to the incredible journey of motherhood. Practice self-compassion and focus on what your body has accomplished rather than unrealistic societal standards.

2. **Mental Health Support**:

Prioritizing mental health is crucial during the postpartum period. Reach out for support from healthcare providers, support groups, or mental health professionals if you're struggling with feelings of sadness, anxiety, or overwhelm. Engage in self-care activities that nourish your mind, body, and soul, such as meditation, journaling, or spending time with loved ones.

By prioritizing core and pelvic floor health, gradually returning to exercise, and practicing self-care and self-compassion, you can navigate the postpartum period with grace and resilience. Remember that every woman's postpartum journey is unique, and it's essential to listen to your body and honor your individual needs as you embark on the path to postpartum fitness and well-being.

Chapter 4: Sample Workouts and Exercise Plans

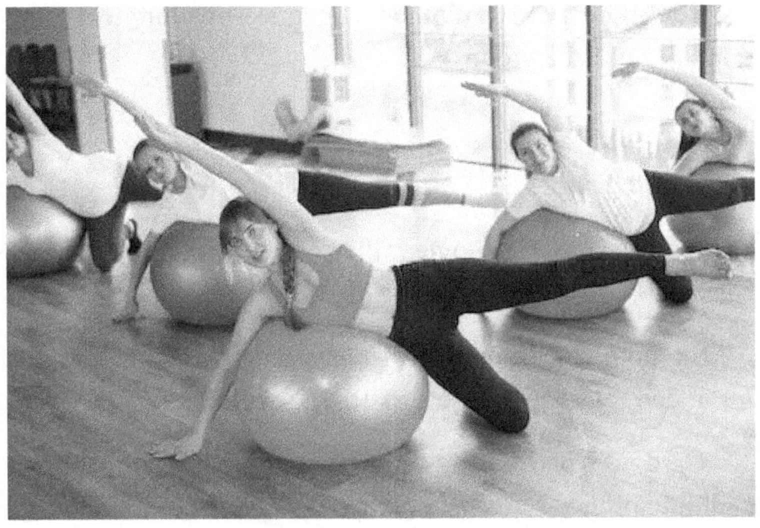

In this chapter, we provide sample prenatal exercise routines tailored to each trimester of pregnancy, as well as postpartum exercise plans designed to support your recovery and gradual return to fitness in the early, mid, and late postpartum periods.

A. **Prenatal Exercise Routines**:

1. **First Trimester:**

- Warm-up: 5-10 minutes of light cardio (e.g., walking or stationary cycling)

- Strength: Bodyweight exercises such as squats, lunges, and modified push-ups (2 sets of 10-12 repetitions)

- Cardio: Low-impact aerobic exercises such as swimming or prenatal yoga (20-30 minutes)

- Cool-down: 5-10 minutes of gentle stretching focusing on major muscle groups

2. **Second Trimester**:

- Warm-up: 5-10 minutes of dynamic stretching or light cardio

- Strength: Incorporate resistance bands or light weights for added resistance (2 sets of 10-12 repetitions)

- Cardio: Continue low-impact activities such as brisk walking, prenatal Pilates, or water aerobics (20-30 minutes)

- Core: Perform pelvic tilts, modified planks, and pelvic floor exercises (2 sets of 10-12 repetitions)

- Cool-down: 5-10 minutes of stretching focusing on flexibility and relaxation

3. **Third Trimester**:

- Warm-up: 5-10 minutes of low-intensity cardio or gentle stretching

- Strength: Focus on exercises that support labor preparation, such as squats, pelvic circles, and seated leg lifts (2 sets of 10-12 repetitions)

- Cardio: Opt for activities that reduce joint impact, such as stationary cycling or prenatal water aerobics (15-20 minutes)

- Relaxation: Incorporate deep breathing exercises and prenatal yoga poses to promote relaxation and stress relief

- Cool-down: 5-10 minutes of gentle stretching to relieve muscle tension and promote flexibility

B. **Postpartum Exercise Plans**:

1. **Early Postpartum (0-6 weeks):**

- Gentle Movement: Begin with short walks or gentle stretches to promote circulation and aid in recovery (10-15 minutes)

- Pelvic Floor Exercises: Perform Kegels and gentle pelvic tilts to strengthen the pelvic floor muscles and aid in bladder control (2 sets of 10-12 repetitions)

- Diaphragmatic Breathing: Practice deep breathing exercises to promote relaxation and reduce stress

- Core Activation: Engage the deep abdominal muscles with pelvic floor contractions and gentle core exercises such as heel slides and pelvic tilts (2 sets of 10-12 repetitions)

2. **Mid-Postpartum (6-12 weeks):**

- Low-Impact Cardio: Gradually increase the duration and intensity of walks or stationary cycling sessions (20-30 minutes)

- Core Strengthening: Progress to more challenging core exercises such as modified planks, bird-dogs, and pelvic bridges (2 sets of 10-12 repetitions)

- Strength Training: Incorporate light resistance training with resistance bands or light weights to build muscle tone and strength (2 sets of 10-12 repetitions)

- Flexibility: Include stretching exercises to improve flexibility and reduce muscle tension (5-10 minutes)

3. **Late Postpartum (12+ weeks):**

- Moderate Cardio: Increase the duration and intensity of cardiovascular activities such as brisk walking, swimming, or low-impact aerobics (30-45 minutes)

- Full-Body Strength Training: Incorporate compound exercises that target multiple muscle groups, such as squats, lunges, and push-ups (2-3 sets of 10-12 repetitions)

- High-Intensity Interval Training (HIIT): Introduce short bursts of high-intensity exercise followed by periods of rest or low-intensity recovery to boost cardiovascular fitness and calorie burn (20-30 minutes)

- Flexibility and Mobility: Prioritize stretching and mobility exercises to maintain range of motion and prevent injury (10-15 minutes)

These sample workouts and exercise plans serve as a starting point for developing a personalized prenatal and postpartum fitness routine. Remember to listen to your body, modify exercises as needed, and consult with your healthcare provider before beginning any new exercise program, especially during the postpartum period. With consistency, patience, and dedication, you can regain strength, improve fitness, and enhance your overall well-being during this transformative time.

Chapter 5: Nutrition and Wellness

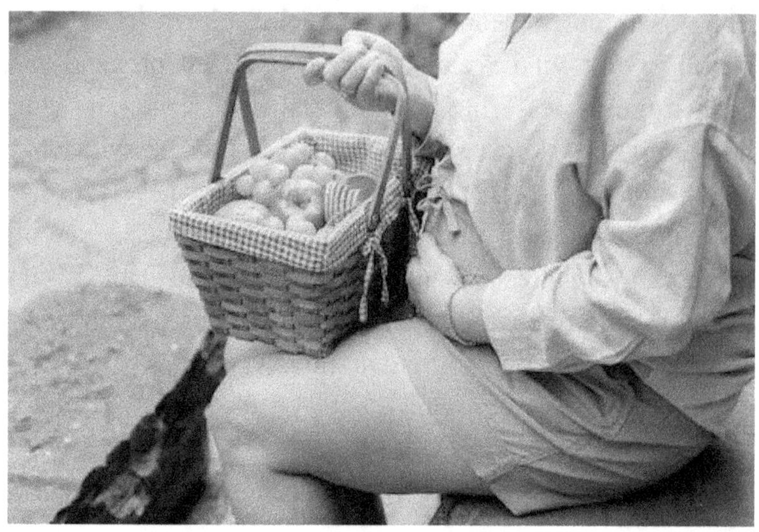

Maintaining a balanced diet and prioritizing overall wellness are essential components of a healthy pregnancy and postpartum journey. In this chapter, we explore the importance of prenatal and postpartum nutrition, strategies for managing sleep and stress, and tips for balancing family life and fitness goals.

A. Prenatal Nutrition:

1. Nutrient Requirements:

During pregnancy, your body requires additional nutrients to support the growth and development of your baby. Focus on consuming a variety of nutrient-dense foods, including fruits, vegetables, whole grains, lean proteins, and healthy fats. Key nutrients to prioritize include folate, iron, calcium, omega-3 fatty acids, and protein, which play critical roles in fetal development and maternal health.

2. **Healthy Eating Tips**:

- Aim for a balanced diet that includes a variety of foods from all food groups.

- Eat small, frequent meals to help manage nausea and maintain steady energy levels.

- Stay hydrated by drinking plenty of water throughout the day.

- Choose whole, unprocessed food whenever possible and limit intake of sugary, high-fat, and processed foods.

- Listen to your body's hunger and fullness cues and eat mindfully to promote healthy eating habits.

B. **Postpartum Nutrition**:

1. **Nutrition for Recovery**:

After childbirth, focus on nourishing your body with nutrient-rich foods to support healing and recovery. Incorporate foods rich in protein, vitamins, and minerals, such as lean meats, fish, fruits, vegetables, whole grains, and dairy products. Stay hydrated and prioritize foods that help replenish nutrients lost during childbirth, such as iron and fluids.

2. **Breastfeeding and Nutrition**:

If you're breastfeeding, your nutritional needs may increase to support milk production and maintain your own health. Aim to eat a well-balanced diet that provides ample calories, protein, and fluids. Incorporate foods known to support lactation, such as oats, flaxseeds, and leafy greens. Consult with a lactation consultant or healthcare provider for personalized guidance on breastfeeding and nutrition.

C. **Sleep and Stress Management**:

Adequate sleep and effective stress management are essential components of overall wellness during pregnancy and postpartum. Prioritize quality sleep by establishing a relaxing bedtime routine, creating a comfortable sleep environment, and practicing relaxation techniques such as deep breathing or meditation. Manage stress through regular exercise, social support, time management strategies, and mindfulness practices.

D. **Balancing Family Life and Fitness Goals**:

Finding a balance between caring for your newborn and prioritizing your own health and fitness goals can be challenging but achievable with careful planning and support. Consider incorporating short, efficient workouts that fit into your schedule, such as home workouts or stroller walks with your baby. Involve your partner, family members, or friends in childcare responsibilities to create time for self-care and exercise. Be flexible and compassionate with yourself as you navigate the demands of parenthood and prioritize your well-being.

By focusing on nutrition, sleep, stress management, and finding balance in family life and fitness goals, you can support your overall wellness during pregnancy and postpartum. Remember to seek support from healthcare providers, family, and friends as needed, and prioritize self-care to nurture both yourself and your growing family.

Chapter 6: Seeking Professional Support

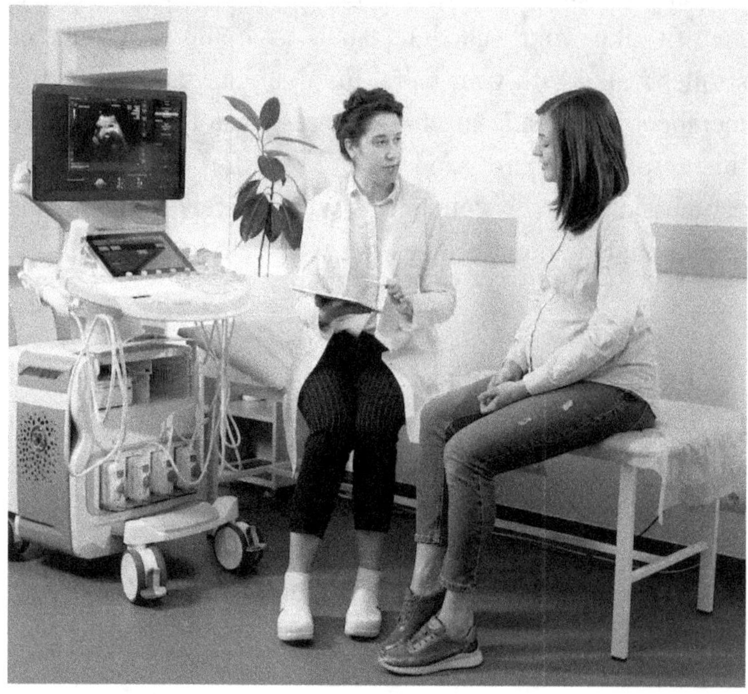

Navigating the complexities of pregnancy and postpartum fitness can be made more manageable with the guidance and support of healthcare providers, fitness specialists, and mental health professionals. In this chapter, we explore the importance of seeking professional support, the role of healthcare providers in your journey, working with personal trainers and fitness specialists, and accessing mental health support for overall well-being.

A. **The Role of Healthcare Providers**:

Your healthcare providers play a crucial role in supporting your pregnancy and postpartum fitness journey. Obstetricians, midwives, and other healthcare professionals can provide personalized guidance and recommendations based on your individual health status, pregnancy-related complications, and fitness goals. They can offer valuable insights into safe exercise practices, monitor your progress throughout pregnancy and postpartum, and address any concerns or medical issues that may arise.

B. **Working with Personal Trainers and Fitness Specialists**:

Personal trainers and fitness specialists with expertise in prenatal and postpartum exercise can offer tailored guidance and support to help you achieve your fitness goals safely and effectively. When selecting a personal trainer or fitness specialist, look for certifications or qualifications in prenatal and postpartum fitness, as well as experience working with pregnant and postpartum clients. A knowledgeable trainer can create customized exercise programs, provide proper form and technique instruction, and offer encouragement and motivation to help you stay on track.

C. **Accessing Mental Health Support**:

Prioritizing mental health is essential during pregnancy and postpartum, as the emotional and psychological aspects of motherhood can significantly impact overall well-being. If you're experiencing feelings of anxiety, depression, or overwhelm, seeking support from mental health professionals can be beneficial. Therapists, counselors, and support groups specializing in perinatal mental health can offer valuable resources, coping strategies, and a safe space to explore your feelings and experiences. Additionally, postpartum support groups and online communities can provide connection, validation, and encouragement from other women who may be facing similar challenges.

By actively seeking professional support from healthcare providers, personal trainers, and mental health professionals, you can enhance your pregnancy and postpartum fitness journey and prioritize your overall health and well-being. Remember that asking for help is a sign of strength, and there are resources and support networks available to assist you every step of the way.

Chapter 7: Real-Life Stories and Testimonials

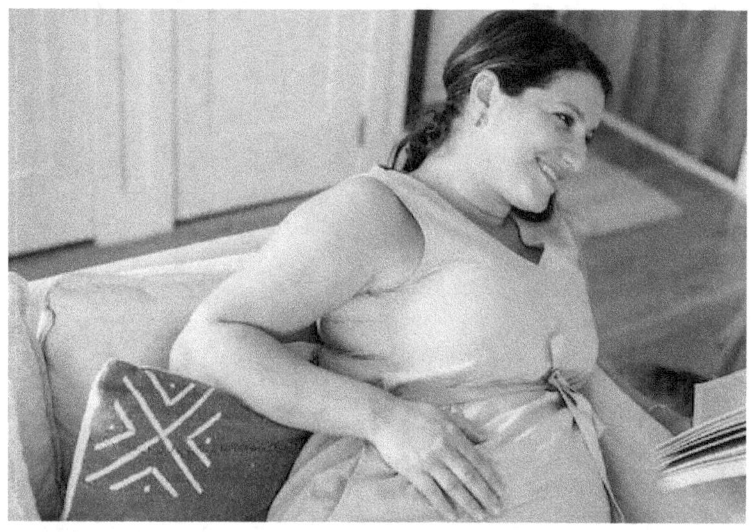

Real-life stories and testimonials offer insight, inspiration, and encouragement to individuals embarking on their pregnancy and postpartum fitness journeys. In this chapter, we share stories of triumph, resilience, and transformation from individuals who have navigated the challenges and celebrated the successes of pregnancy and postpartum fitness.

A. **Personal Stories of Pregnancy and Postpartum Fitness Journeys:**

Each pregnancy and postpartum fitness journey is unique, and hearing personal stories from individuals who have walked similar paths can provide reassurance and solidarity. From first-time mothers to seasoned parents, these stories offer glimpses into the diverse experiences and emotions encountered along the way. Whether it's overcoming physical limitations, navigating mental health challenges, or celebrating milestones, these personal narratives highlight the strength, resilience, and beauty of the human spirit.

B. **Overcoming Challenges**:

Pregnancy and postpartum fitness journeys are not without their challenges. From physical discomfort and fatigue to emotional ups and downs, individuals often face obstacles that test their resolve and determination. In this section, we explore the various challenges encountered during pregnancy and postpartum and the strategies employed to overcome them. Whether it's finding creative ways to stay active despite physical limitations, seeking support from healthcare providers and loved ones, or cultivating resilience in the face of setbacks, these stories illustrate the power of perseverance and adaptation in the pursuit of fitness and wellness.

C. **Success Stories**:

Amidst the challenges and obstacles, there are countless stories of success and triumph in the realm of pregnancy and postpartum fitness. In this section, we celebrate the achievements, milestones, and victories of individuals who have embraced fitness as an integral part of their journey to motherhood. From regaining strength and mobility after childbirth to achieving personal fitness goals and milestones, these success stories inspire hope, motivation, and determination. They serve as reminders that with dedication, perseverance, and support, it is possible to thrive physically, mentally, and emotionally during the transformative journey of pregnancy and postpartum.

By sharing real-life stories and testimonials, we aim to uplift, inspire, and empower individuals as they embark on their own pregnancy and postpartum fitness journeys. These narratives remind us that we are not alone in our experiences and that through shared struggles and triumphs, we can find strength, connection, and community.

Conclusion:

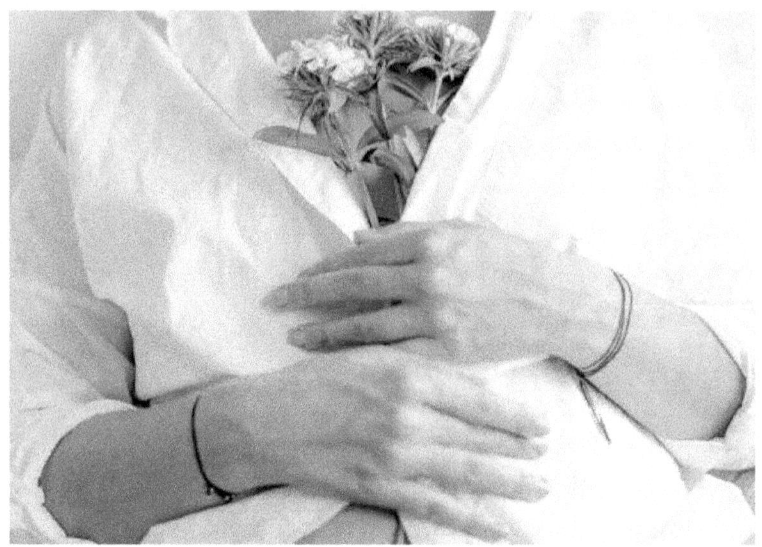

As you reach the conclusion of "Pregnancy and Postpartum Fitness," it's essential to reflect on the transformative journey you've embarked upon and look ahead to the possibilities that lie ahead. In this final chapter, we offer encouragement, inspiration, and practical tips to support you as you continue your journey toward healthy pregnancy and postpartum fitness.

A. **The Journey Continues**:

The journey of pregnancy and postpartum fitness is not a destination but a continuous evolution. As you transition through different stages of motherhood, your fitness needs and goals may evolve, presenting new opportunities for growth and self-discovery. Embrace each step of the journey with an open heart and a willingness to learn and adapt. Remember that every challenge you face and every triumph you celebrate is a testament to your strength, resilience, and dedication to your health and well-being.

B. **Encouragement and Inspiration**:

Throughout the pages of this book, you've encountered stories of triumph, resilience, and transformation from individuals who have navigated the complexities of pregnancy and postpartum fitness. Draw inspiration from their experiences and use their stories as fuel to propel you forward on your journey. Remember that you are capable of overcoming obstacles, achieving your goals, and embracing the beauty of motherhood with confidence and grace.

C. **Final Tips for Healthy Pregnancy and Postpartum Fitness**:

As you continue your pregnancy and post-partum fitness journey, keep the following tips in mind to support your health and well-being:

1. Listen to your body: Trust your intuition and listen to your body's cues. If something doesn't feel right, modify or pause your exercise routine and consult with your healthcare provider.

2. Prioritize self-care: Make time for self-care activities that nourish your body, mind, and soul. Whether it's taking a bubble bath, practicing meditation, or enjoying a healthy meal, prioritizing activities that promote relaxation and rejuvenation.

3. Stay connected: Seek support from your healthcare providers, family, friends, and fellow mothers. Surround yourself with a supportive network of individuals who uplift and encourage you on your journey.

4. Celebrate your progress: Celebrate every milestone, no matter how small. Whether it's completing a workout, reaching a fitness goal, or simply finding moments of joy amidst the challenges of motherhood, take time to acknowledge and celebrate your achievements.

As you close the pages of this book and embark on the next chapter of your journey, remember that you are not alone. You have the knowledge, tools, and support to navigate the challenges and embrace the joys of pregnancy and postpartum fitness. With determination, resilience, and a commitment to your well-being, you can thrive physically, mentally, and emotionally as you embrace the transformative journey of motherhood.

45

About The Author

Eric Uroh is a passionate advocate for health and well-being. With a deep concern for the overall wellness of individuals, Eric has dedicated his life to helping others achieve their health goals and lead happier, more fulfilling lives.

As a fervent fitness enthusiast, Eric Uroh brings a wealth of personal experience and knowledge to the realm of weight loss and healthy living. They have spent countless hours researching, experimenting with various strategies, and engaging in physical activities to discover what truly works for achieving and maintaining a healthy weight. This firsthand experience has given Eric Uroh unique insights into the challenges and triumphs that individuals face on their weight loss journeys.

Eric's unwavering commitment to health and well-being shines through in their writing, coaching, and advocacy work. They believe that everyone has the potential to transform their lives through informed choices and dedicated effort. Through this book, Eric shares his expertise, offering readers a practical and comprehensive guide to achieving their weight loss goals and embracing a healthier and happier lifestyle.

Join Eric Uroh on this transformative journey toward better health and discover the strategies and inspiration you need to embark on your path to success. Your goals are within reach, and Eric is here to guide you every step of the way.

Books By This Author

Title: Fitness Motivation and Goal Setting

Description:

Your Comprehensive Guide to Achieving Lasting Results and Transforming Your Life

Are you ready to embark on a transformative journey towards a healthier, stronger, and more vibrant you? "Fitness Motivation and Goal Setting" is your comprehensive guide to unlocking your full potential for lifelong health and wellness.

This eBook is your trusted companion on the path to fitness success, offering a roadmap that combines the power of motivation and effective goal setting. Inside, you'll discover the secrets to igniting and sustaining your motivation, setting smart and achievable fitness goals, and crafting a personalized fitness plan tailored to your unique needs and aspirations.

With practical insights, expert advice, and real-life success stories, you'll explore the art of overcoming obstacles, building resilience, and staying motivated throughout your journey. Dive into motivational techniques, harness the power of visualization, and learn the importance of accountability and support systems that will keep you on track.

As you progress through the chapters, you'll find inspiration in the stories of individuals who have already achieved remarkable fitness transformations. Discover the strategies that worked for them and apply these lessons to your journey.

To equip you further, we've curated a valuable toolkit of resources and tools, including recommended apps, websites, fitness-tracking tools, books, podcasts, and online communities, ensuring you have the support you need every step of the way.

Your fitness journey is a lifelong adventure, and "Fitness Motivation and Goal Setting" is your trusted guide. Whether you're just starting or looking to revitalize your fitness routine, this eBook will empower you to set and achieve your goals, maintain momentum, and embrace a healthier, more fulfilling life. Begin your journey today and unlock the boundless potential within you. Your transformation starts now.

Title: Weight Loss Strategies

Description:

Unlock the Secrets to Sustainable Weight Loss and a Healthier You!

Are you tired of fad diets and quick fixes that don't deliver lasting results? Are you looking for a comprehensive guide to achieving your weight loss goals while improving your overall well-being? Look no further! "Weight Loss Strategies" is your ultimate resource for embarking on a transformative journey to a healthier and happier life.

Inside this eBook, you'll discover a wealth of knowledge and practical strategies that will empower you to take control of your weight and achieve sustainable results. Say goodbye to the cycle of yo-yo dieting and hello to a balanced, healthier lifestyle.

Here's what you can expect to find within these pages:

- The Science Behind Weight Loss: Understand the fundamentals of weight loss, from caloric deficits to metabolism and body composition. Gain the knowledge you need to make informed choices.

- Nutrition and Diet: Learn the art of healthy eating with insights into balanced diets, portion control, and mindful eating. Explore effective dietary plans, including low-carb diets, the Mediterranean diet, and intermittent fasting.

- Exercise and Physical Activity: Discover the importance of exercise in weight loss and explore various types of physical activities, from cardiovascular workouts to strength training and flexibility exercises. Create a personalized workout plan and learn how to stay consistent with your exercise routines.

- Lifestyle and Behavior Modification: Cultivate healthy habits for weight loss success, including the importance of sleep, stress management, and hydration. Break bad habits such as smoking and excessive alcohol consumption, and build a supportive environment with the help of family and friends or accountability partners.

- Monitoring and Tracking Progress: Unlock the power of progress tracking with insights into why it's crucial to monitor your weight and measurements. Keep a food journal, utilize technology and apps, and adjust your strategies based on your results.

- Dealing with Plateaus and Setbacks: Overcome common hurdles like weight loss plateaus with effective strategies. Learn how to handle setbacks and relapses while maintaining unwavering motivation during challenging times.

- Weight Maintenance: Successfully transition from weight loss to maintenance, develop a sustainable lifestyle, prevent weight regain, and celebrate your achievements and milestones.

In "Weight Loss Strategies," you'll find evidence-based guidance, practical tips, and expert advice to help you navigate the complexities of weight loss. Whether you're a beginner just starting your journey or someone looking to refine their approach, this eBook is your comprehensive roadmap to a healthier, happier life.

Don't wait any longer to take control of your weight and well-being. Get started on your path to success with "Weight Loss Strategies" today! Your transformation begins here.

Title: Healthy Cooking

Description:

Are you ready to embark on a culinary journey that will transform the way you approach food and nourish your body? "Healthy Cooking 101" is your comprehensive guide to a more vibrant, balanced, and health-conscious lifestyle through the art of cooking.

In this thoughtfully crafted eBook, you will explore the fundamental principles of healthy cooking, from understanding nutritional basics to mastering cooking techniques that preserve nutrients and enhance flavors. Discover how to plan well-balanced meals that incorporate lean proteins, whole grains, and an abundance of vegetables and fruits.

"Healthy Cooking" caters to a wide range of dietary needs and preferences, offering guidance on weight management, heart health, diabetes management, allergies, sensitivities, and even vegetarian and vegan cooking. With a focus on quality ingredients, you'll learn how to create delicious and nutritious recipes for breakfast, lunch, dinner, snacks, desserts, and beverages.

But this eBook goes beyond the kitchen. It delves into the holistic aspects of healthy living, helping you integrate exercise, manage stress, and make ethical food choices that align with your values. Explore how mindful eating and social connections enrich your relationship with food.

As you journey through the pages of "Healthy Cooking," you'll gain valuable insights into overcoming common challenges, staying on track with your goals, seeking support and accountability, and celebrating your successes.

Whether you're a seasoned home cook or just beginning to explore the joys of the kitchen, this eBook provides you with the knowledge, inspiration, and practical tools to make healthy cooking a sustainable and rewarding part of your life. Take the first step toward a healthier, happier you and embark on a culinary adventure that nourishes both body and soul. Your future of flavorful, nutritious meals starts here.

Title: Fitness for Busy Professionals

Description:

In the fast-paced world of modern professionals, finding time for fitness amidst the demands of a career can seem like an insurmountable challenge. Yet, maintaining a healthy lifestyle is essential for thriving in both personal and professional spheres. "Fitness for Busy Professionals" is a comprehensive guide tailored specifically for individuals navigating the intricate balance between career ambitions and well-being.

This eBook delves into the unique challenges faced by busy professionals, from time constraints and mental exhaustion to sedentary lifestyles and limited resources. It offers practical strategies and time-saving tips for integrating fitness into even the busiest of schedules, empowering readers to prioritize their health without sacrificing professional success.

From mindful scheduling and micro-workouts to leveraging technology and incorporating stress management techniques, this eBook provides actionable insights to help busy professionals overcome obstacles and establish sustainable fitness routines. Each chapter is packed with valuable information, actionable steps, and real-world examples to guide readers on their journey to improved health and vitality.

With a focus on cultivating a positive mindset, setting realistic goals, and celebrating progress, "Fitness for Busy Professionals" equips readers with the tools and motivation needed to make lasting lifestyle changes. It emphasizes the importance of self-care, encourages individuals to prioritize their well-being amidst career demands, and empowers them to take control of their health journey.

Whether you're a CEO with a packed schedule or an entrepreneur juggling multiple projects, this eBook is your roadmap to achieving fitness success during a hectic professional life. Let "Fitness for Busy Professionals" be your guide as you embark on a journey towards improved health, increased energy, and enhanced productivity. It's time to invest in yourself and unlock your full potential because a healthier, happier you is the key to thriving in every aspect of your life.

Title: Healthy Aging

Description:

"Healthy Aging" is a comprehensive guide to thriving as you grow older, filled with practical advice, evidence-based strategies, and inspiring insights to help you live your best life in your later years.

In this eBook, you'll discover:

- Expert tips for staying physically active, eating well, and maintaining overall health as you age.

- Insights into understanding the biological changes, common health concerns, and psychological aspects of aging.

- Strategies for incorporating physical activity into your daily routine, overcoming barriers to exercise, and staying fit at any age.

- Guidance on the importance of nutrition, dietary recommendations, meal planning, and addressing nutritional challenges in older age.

- Practical advice for maintaining mental and emotional well-being, reducing stress, fostering social connections, and keeping your mind sharp.

- Tips for preventive health measures, including regular check-ups, vaccinations, managing chronic conditions, and promoting good sleep hygiene.

- Lifestyle factors for healthy aging, such as maintaining a healthy weight, managing chronic conditions, limiting alcohol consumption, and embracing relaxation techniques.

- Guidance on adapting to life transitions, planning for the future, and creating a support network to navigate the challenges and opportunities of aging.

Whether you're approaching retirement, already enjoying your golden years, or caring for aging loved ones, "Healthy Aging" is your essential companion for aging gracefully, embracing vitality, and living life to the fullest.

www.ingramcontent.com/pod-product-compliance
Lightning Source LLC
Chambersburg PA
CBHW071000250726
48663CB00002B/306